Biofrequencies
and
Parkinson's Disease

I0439437

SHARRY EDWARDS: For many years we did not know how we were making this progress. We only knew we had results. One of the things Dr. <u>John Apsley</u> and I had been talking about is the idea that we are influencing the harmonic resonance, the magnetic potential of the body. That is how we are helping people heal themselves. We started running some tests and sure enough, it seems like we are changing the magnetic potential of the frequencies of the cells. So now that we have that underlying answer.

One of the things that Dr. John Apsley said, which sort of blew me away, was: "Sharry's work defines and demonstrates the unifying field theory that defied Einstein". He said, "We know that you're changing the electrical potential". It's like

Biofrequencies and Parkinsons Disease

some of Stan Tennant's work where he goes in and puts a different electrical charge on a cell or some of Bjorn Nordenstrom's work where he puts a charge on a tumor and the cancer cells just dry up. If it's a positive cell charge - like a 30 - he puts a negative 30 on it and then the tumor just goes away. Dr. Apsley is thinking that is how we are getting the results that we are getting but we are using a computer program which tells us what frequencies to use, what formulations to use, how to put them together, what's the priority and that shows what is really going on.

We have now done probably more than 30 but less than 50 Parkinson's client evaluations. We are finding that Parkinson's is just a throw-away diagnosis. When they don't know what else to call it, they're just going to throw in Parkinson's as a diagnosis. We can begin to look at this and see that many of these cell signaling problems come from *the inability to use glutamate. In conjunction, it can come from an inability to use cholesterol or low testosterone or unbalanced lKrebs cycle or low vitamin C or issues with trimethylglycine. It is coming from so many directions I don't think conventional medicine really knows what this disease is. They are just lumping a lot of people together that have similar symptoms but very different root causes.*

What causes of Parkinson's disease have you now been able to identify?

SHARRY EDWARDS: There are three or four biggies. There are two major enzymes. One is called COMT and that stands for Catechol-O-methyl transferase. It is a genetic issue; an enzyme that degrades catecholamines like dopamine, epinephrine and norepinephrine. It is actually an issue in the gene. People can read more about this at www.heartfixer.com. The other one is Aromatic l-amino acid decarboxylase, but that one has another name which makes much more sense for Parkinson's people: it is also known as _tryptophan decarboxylase_. Tryptophan is intimately involved in the whole pathway to making L-dopa and dopamine. One of the things that trips people up with that is potassium. The other part that trips people up is B3 - niacin.

We have found a tremendous toxin load involved with Parkinson's. The software we designed is able to identify the frequency correlates of the toxins. Many of them have a base in _chlordane_ and that was outlawed in the United States a decade or so ago. If people have the kind of Parkinson's that shrivels up their hands and the hands look atrophied, chlordane or a similar herbicide is usually involved. It is used on pot (marijuana). It is still being used in other countries. They used it a lot in the 50's and 60's on tomatoes and a lot of different kinds of vegetables. Looking at the effects of those toxins we are seeing that the body is just breaking *down and is not able to rebuild itself.*

Another one we found was the inability to use <u>*methionine*</u> *and its required cofactor* <u>*glutathione*</u>*. The third one is a combination of* <u>*glutamic acid*</u> *and glutamate and all of that comes into play* <u>*with Genetically Modified foods*</u> *(GMOs), particularly anything that contains* <u>*gluten*</u> *like oats, rye, barley and wheat.*

There are three or four biggies that we see BioAcoustically. One of the biggest ones that started out with somebody who came from your show was <u>*radiation poisoning*</u>*. We're going back and looking at things from* <u>*Chernobyl*</u> *and even farther back to nuclear plants and finding out that radiation poisoning is another form of toxicity that is causing Parkinson's and cancer. It robs the body of its electrical force so the body is in a constant state of stress in its attempt to get rid of free radical damage. The body gets overwhelmed because the cells work hard* *enough taking care of the damage. Right now we are seeing high levels of radiation in the milk and the water and the grass and the hay and the feeds and the air.*

We are following some people who have exposure to radiation coming from Fukushima. Their nervous systems have begun to break down. That is another cause of Parkinson's. The sheathing surrounding the nerves does not get nourished and replenished. The cell signaling system becomes impaired and eventually breaks down. We have created a computer program to identify this. It sounds very difficult. It sounds like a lot of information but the computer program will separate it out and say okay, this is the root cause.

Did the people who had radiation exposure live in the United States?

SHARRY EDWARDS: Yes. Marian can tell us about the issues she has had from having been exposed to radiation from her job at a nuclear energy plant.

MARIAN LEWIS: I was at the end of my line watching my life ebb away. I cannot tolerate the Parkinson's medications. I was losing weight and just literally wasting away. I had been diagnosed almost two years ago. I started out on the meds, had problems and then they got me adjusted. I did okay for a while, but then I started having major problems and just could not function.

We were planning to make a trip north. We live in Florida. I am a 74-year old grandmother and this was going to be my goodbye trip to my family because I just felt that I was dying. I just happened to hear your radio show and Sharry Edwards was on that day. I just knew I had to go there. So I asked my husband if he would mind making a 700 mile detour. He agreed and I thank God for that because it has given me my life back. Not only did it help me with my Parkinson's symptoms

Biofrequencies and Parkinsons Disease

but many other issues that I have.

Now, I have taken the training to become a BioAcoustic practitioner. I was in Sharry's office and she said, "Oh my, you have so many issues, we really need to get you to a practitioner, but we don't have any in Florida". There I was and in my weakened condition, I said, "You're looking at her". She said "fine". I thought she might tell me that I was too old or too weak or whatever, but she didn't. She encouraged me and I did the training on-line after I got home from my trip. I survived the class.

I just got all my equipment this afternoon and I'm ready to go. I've got people lined up and I want to specialize in Parkinson's. I've got so many Parkinson's friends here. At the time I said I was going to do this, I had no idea if I could physically or financially do it. But here I am and doing better every day.

Biofrequencies and Parkinsons Disease

I have to tell you that my story began when I was 18 when I was exposed to radioactive material. We worked in a uranium processing plant in Southwestern Pennsylvania that is now buried under 20 feet of earth with a barbed wire fence around it. I did not tell Sharry that I was exposed to this, but she found it in my voice print after all those years. At age 23, I developed a low thyroid problem. At age 37, I had cancer in the saliva gland and I had radical surgery on the left side of my face that took my facial nerve. The left side of my face is paralyzed. When I turned 50, 14 years later, I had lung cancer. The same cancer returned. Then at age 71, I started with a little tremor that they diagnosed a year later as Parkinson's disease.

It all stems back from being exposed to radiation. This is my fear of what's going to happen to our babies; our children and our grandchildren, only it's going to happen much earlier to them. I really feel

Biofrequencies and Parkinsons Disease

we have the ability to do something about it. We need to get the knowledge out there. I had some wonderful experiences with Sharry.

While she was doing my tones the first day, I felt tingling sensations. My left foot was turned in and my toes were curled under when I went to her. That night after the initial treatment my toes straightened out. The next day, I noticed some feeling, a strange sensation on my left side where the drainage tube had been from my lung surgery. The feeling was coming back. There had been a numb spot there. There was also a little tingling feeling in the side of my face, which had been paralyzed for 37 years. Now, I have slight movement in my face. My nerves are regenerating. I was getting zingers all over the place and a burning sensation in my nose.

The following day after we left Sharry's clinic we went through Pennsylvania and stopped for gasoline. As I came out of the restroom and approached our car, I said, "Oh my goodness, I smell gasoline!" My husband said, "Well, I'm filling the car." I said, "No, no, no, I smell it!" He said, "Oh my goodness!" We got to my daughter's house the next day and my grandson had made popcorn and I smelled it!

The following day, I went to the grocery store. Now the last time I had been to a grocery store, I couldn't even make it around the store. I had to use a wheelchair. But, here I was walking around the store swinging my arms unassisted and smelling all sorts of things in the store. I saw a pile of cantaloupe and I decided to test it. I went over and I remembered my grandmother saying, "You could tell a good cantaloupe if you could smell it". So I thought it would be my dumb luck to pick up one that's not ripe. But, I picked one up, put it to my nose and I could smell it and honestly, I sobbed over the darn cantaloupe. I could not speak.

Biofrequencies and Parkinsons Disease

My husband came running over saying, "What is wrong! Did someone say something to upset you?" I said, "No, no, no. I can smell it! I can smell the cantaloupe!" It was just a wonderful thing. For seven years, I hadn't smelled anything and now in just a few days, my sense of smell had returned.

I still have Parkinson's issues that I'm dealing with, but as Sharry said I have to "peel the onion one layer at a time" because I have many, many issues. I developed a heart problem as well, but it's all related. The thyroid started, then the heart and the cancer and the Parkinson's, they're all related to radiation exposure and that's why I just really feel that it's so important for people to be aware and get on board. We can find out what's happening and learn how to fix these things. We have to help ourselves because the conventional medical doctors can't help us. They can only give us more drugs and they just don't work for everyone. I still have some tremor but it's diminished quite a bit and at times it isn't there. I'm still working on it. I noticed an improvement in my face just today. I looked in a mirror and I saw a little jiggling in my chin and also under my left eye.

The feeling has returned. The whole side of my face was numb. It was like when you have Novocain. I would often bite the inside of my cheek and not realize it. Now, I have total feeling inside and outside of my face. Everyone says I look different. I really think that the deep depression that I had on the side of my face may be starting to fill in a little bit. It seems like it's not as deep as it was. I don't know if there's tissue growing back there or what, but it's a fascinating thing.

SHARRY EDWARDS: Marian's a very determined lady and I think that helps with her case too. But to be able to identify the frequencies of a patient's foot and watch the foot relax, we can say – here are the B vitamins that are causing her tremor and here is the cholesterol issue - to have that available and watch people get so excited about finally having a definitive answer is awesome. It is more than excitement. It is exhuberation. It is like jumping up and saying, "Oh, look at my foot!" I've just never gotten over that delight and seeing people not in pain or being able to use their hand again. I want this kind of technique to be available to everybody.

Are you going to sponsor a class on bio-frequencies in Florida?

MARIAN LEWIS: I've got people who are taking numbers in my Parkinson's support group. They are so excited; people who are in their 70s and 80s who want a better life. They don't want to be zombies. Most of them were men who were very successful in their lives and they've become like zombies. It's so sad.

Biofrequencies and Parkinsons Disease

I found a wonderful Parkinson's movement disorder doctor who is just floored by all of this. He doesn't know what to think of me. I keep sending him more and more patients, around 20 so far. I told a few of them who had seen a regular Neurologist, not a Movement Disorder Specialist, "I don't think you have Parkinson's disease. Go see my doctor for a second opinion." One of the ladies I sent came back to me and said, "You know your doctor said I don't Parkinson's disease?" He said, "Oh darn, that woman was right again!" The woman's problem was caused by a combination of drugs for other issues she had.

There's something more to this Parkinson's thing than what they would have us believe. Before you know what you have you go to see a doctor who is not a movement disorder specialist. They have you walk up and down the hall and do a couple of things with your hand and five minutes later, out of the blue, they say "You have Parkinson's Disease. It's a degenerative disease. Take these pills. There is nothing we can do. I'll see you in three or four months and then I'll give you some more pills until you can't take those pills anymore because you're going to get worse." It's just awful.

When I insisted that there had to be something that I could do, they sent me to physical therapy for a few weeks. On the second day, a young perky girl came in and she showed me a Mercedes-top-of-the-line walker. At that time, I was sometimes falling and freezing. I was doing all those things I don't do anymore and I said, "Who are you talking to girl, you're not talking to me. I noticed you said when I need it, not if I need it!" I just wasn't prepared for that. I refuse to lie down and die. I mean, I've been through a lot already and I'm just not going to lie down and die. I always told my husband, "A disease will not kill me, the cure will." I say this because I am so sensitive to drugs and the side effects are terrible.

SHARRY EDWARDS: Marian, one of the very first things I noticed when you were here is that you could just pop up and down out of the chair when you couldn't do that before. That was our first indicator that this was working for you.

Marian: Yes, getting in and out of the car, out of the chair, and walking by myself.

SHARRY EDWARDS: This is not a one-time deal. It is not something that can be done over the phone. There are people that are getting very upset with us when they call here and say, "Can you give me some information about why I have Parkinson's?" Then I say, "Yes I can." We can look at their nutrition and their genes and other things, but when they want me to cure them over the phone, that's just not how this works. We do have some practitioners who will travel. What happened to Marian could not have happened had she not at least come to our research office in the beginning. You see it for yourself and you experience it. That is what makes it real. That is what convinces you about what is going on.

MARIAN LEWIS: You're right. It takes time. I'm still working on the tremor. It is less than it was and I'm not on the medication. It is a process and you have to be patient.

Describe for us what happened when you came to Sharry Edwards' clinic.

MARIAN LEWIS: They took some pictures of me and some video. They asked me what I expected. They asked me what my reason was for coming there and I had to fill out some papers. It wasn't long before Sharry took me into her office and put a microphone in front of me. I had to speak into the microphone for about 30 seconds or so.

First we talked about my health and then I talked about our trip. She wanted me to talk about my symptoms, but it becomes almost routine because you repeat the same thing to every doctor and every person. Then she wanted something that was spontaneous, so we talked about the trip. She took the voice prints and came back and started to use some tones. I took them back to the hotel that night in a tone box and listened to them that evening and returned the next day.

I was overzealous. I wanted a cure and I wanted it yesterday. I listened to the tones constantly and overdosed on some of the things just like you can on medication. I had listened to them too long. I had them on from the time I left as much as I could. I had it on all night. That was not the instruction, but I thought more is better. I was just too anxious and I had to be adjusted. When we left, I understood more after they explained the procedure again. You know you hear what you want to hear. Even though they had written it down, I still decided I knew better, but I didn't know better.

Describe the ToneBox for us.

MARIAN LEWIS: You have headphones. It is a box about the size of a pack of cigarettes with some buttons on it. My husband was also very skeptical. He thought this was a dying wish kind of thing so he took me there and put up with me. Sharry asked him, "Wouldn't you like to have your vocal analysis done too?" He said okay and I almost fainted. He had gone through 45 radiation treatments of prostate cancer and he has diabetes. He had a shoulder issue where he couldn't reach around to get his wallet out of his back pocket. We thought that was psychological but it apparently wasn't.

We shared the same ToneBox; they put the tones in the box for both of us. It wasn't long before he was able to reach in his back pocket. That wasn't something that he had told the practitioner when he went there. Sharry did not do his tones. Another gal that worked with her did his while Sharry was doing mine. I don't even think he told her that he had that problem, but it was no longer a problem after a few days. He went to the doctor here just last week and so far he's doing very well with his numbers on his prostate and his diabetes and so forth. His symptoms were not as visible as mine, of course, because Parkinson's has very visible symptoms.

Everybody says to me, "Oh you look different" or they go to help me when I don't need help anymore. They stand in awe and wonderment, "How did you do that?" They say, "We know you pray but we didn't know you had that kind of connection."

SHARRY EDWARDS: We tested Marian every step of the way. When we were presenting sounds for the tremors we had her hold out a piece of paper until we found the tone that made the tremor stop. When we were working on her foot we worked with her feet and her standing up and walking. Every little piece that we did we were checking ourselves. We loan people the ToneBox overnight to make sure this is going to work because we don't want people to buy something that's not going to work for them. Most people come from a long, long way. When we take the voice we look at the frequencies of the voice. We look at the harmonics. We look at the distance between the tones. I used to do all of this by hand and just with my hearing but now we've developed computer programs so that everybody can do this. This is not some special talent you have to have to be able to take this vocal print and put it into the computer and get your report.

MARIAN LEWIS: I can even do it. I had some computer background but only self-taught. I have a high school diploma. I have no biology nor chemistry knowledge.

Biofrequencies and Parkinsons Disease

I find that when I talk to people about doing this, they feel that they have to have some kind of degree in something. I encourage people to take the training no matter what your age or even your condition. It is an intense course, but if you can sit there long enough, do it. I did collapse at the end of the day. I have to say that. I went 9:00 to 5:00 or 9:00 to 6:00 with the class, did homework and then I crashed. A few weeks ago I couldn't even walk across my living room floor, so I thought that was just marvelous.

> **Was it your intention to enroll in the biofrequencies classes when you went to see Sharry Edwards?**

MARIAN LEWIS: I was barely able to function. I just felt like God was leading me there to tell you the truth. I really felt the whole thing was part of a master plan that I needed to go there, that I was supposed to be there. There was a reason for it all. There was something more that I needed to do with my life. It has literally turned me around because I felt like I was dying. And, I've never felt like that even when I was 37 and told I had less than 10% chance to live when I had cancer of the saliva gland. Nor, even when I was told that I had less than two years to live when I was 50 and I had lung cancer. I just couldn't believe that I could live anymore. It wasn't the Parkinson's itself. It was the medications that were making me so sick that I thought I was dying.

We need to blast this information out to the world. We need to get more people trained. I hope to be Sound Health Options representative here in Florida for Parkinson's disease. There are a lot of other senior ailments that I'll be dealing with I know because that's just the senior people that I'm around and with all of the time. But we need to deal with the younger ones too. I have grandchildren with ADD and ADHD and bi-polar syndrome. All of these things can be addressed and taken care of. We need to

Biofrequencies and Parkinsons Disease

get more people involved.

Is this treatment like taking medicine?

MARIAN LEWIS: Oh it's better than that. I call it sound hope. I'm very active in the Hope Parkinson's Program *here in Southwest Florida. It's a wonderful program that has helped me so much. They have free exercise and balance classes, water aerobics, dance, art, music and almost anything you can think of including Yoga and Tai Chi type exercises specifically for Parkinson's people. They have numerous support groups for patients and caregivers. In the wintertime our numbers triple, so I have been asked to speak at several of the Parkinson's support groups this fall and winter. They want to hear about sound BioAcoustics and what it can do for them. I want people to be aware of this radiation threat because it is real and it is damaging. People need to join the* Guardian Network *[www.GuardiansOfThePeople.com] and be a part of that.*

How do Bio-Frequencies work?

SHARRY EDWARDS: You have a brain which is your central processing unit. All the signals from the brain go out to the rest of the body through your neural network. We just found a way to tap in to that system. If Marian, for example, is not getting a signal to her toe, we can give her brain a signal that feeds her toe or give her brain a signal that feeds the dopamine pathway and that addresses whatever is going on. We are tapping into the energy system of the body.

I don't think this is a new medicine. It is a very old medicine. This is how people knew how to cure themselves in the beginning. The aborigines still do it with sound and rhythm. This is what the <u>Templars</u> *did in the 14th Century. So, new medicine? Advanced medicine? Star Trek medicine? Old medicine? Indian medicine? It's all of those. Is frequency our new medicine or an ancient mystery revealed? I think it is both.*

© *Parkinsons Recovery* 26

Biofrequencies and Parkinsons Disease

If people want to see some of those articles they can go to our website http://www.SoundHealthOptions.com and read the research articles. One of the things we are finding with Parkinson's is that it is just not the Parkinson's. It's allergies. It's methylation (how people use their incoming resources). It's dystonia. It's spasticity. It's inflammation. It's radiation exposure. It's tetanus exposure. It's several things at once. Our goal is to have at least one Parkinson's trained person in every state and every province in Canada.

What is the Guardian Network?

SHARRY EDWARDS: This has been going on for about little over a year. Every month we meet as a group: Guardians of the People. This month we focused on the immune system and exposed people to the immune system software program. Tones that are biggies for the immune system are F, F-sharp and A-sharp. We provide software programs for the Guardians each month. We teach them how to evaluate allergies or Parkinson's or losing weight or building muscle or whatever they'd like. With the immune system there are a lot of magnesium and cholesterol issues so they can do their own evaluation. We give them the information about what they should be looking for. That is the free part.

We sell the computer programs for $185 dollars each. If you join the Guardian Network – meaning you are someone who will commit to taking this information to the community – the computer program is $40.

We are talking about doing a workshop particularly for people with Parkinson's. If anyone wants to be a part of this program - and it's on line- they can learn to do this now. We are going to provide some scholarship funds to help people take the course and be that one person that is providing information in an area. I envision Marian having two or three other people trained to help her out because she's going to have more work than she can possibly do. We are not going to restrict it totally to one person per state, but we'd like to see at least one person per state join us in this effort.

Is it necessary for a person to attend your onsite training program for the entire week?

SHARRY EDWARDS: They can do it online. Marian did it online.

MARIAN LEWIS: Yes, I did it online because I didn't think I could physically go back again. I really was not very strong when I did it. I was able to do it in my own home. It's a lot of work; it's a lot of information.

SHARRY EDWARDS: We have an annual conference to provide people all the new information. This year we are providing a way for people to do their own blood test by taking a vocal profile and looking at every aspect of their blood just as if they sent it off to the lab and paid seven or eight thousand dollars. That's the biggie. This is medicine for the people – that's why we're calling it Guardians of the People

How does a person find a local BioAcoustic practitioner?

SHARRY EDWARDS: You will find a map and a list of practitioners by clicking on the "Clinical Service" and the "Find a Practitioner" links on our website. The list is rotated every few months because people get run over with having too much business and they can't handle it. A lot of bio-frequency practitioners send somebody else to be trained as an assistant to them. That's a far smaller course, a one-day course.

Tell us about Happy Hour

SHARRY EDWARDS: We have happy hour every other Tuesday. It is from 6 to 7 Eastern Time, so that's 3 to 4 Pacific Time. It is free. For information or an invitation just go to: www.SoundHealthOptions.com/happy_hour.html. The Happy Hour link looks like a little postage stamp on the right-hand side of the page. Click that link and you will see how to join us for Happy Hour. We have 30 to 40 people usually. The first people with their hand up usually get to have an analysis done that day, on-line, for free.

Last night we did a Parkinson's case. We found out several things from doing the analysis. We found there was a genetic issue with enzymes. There was an inability to use trimethylglycine and there was a chlordane-based toxin. He did have the atrophied hands which he reported to us when I said, "Based on what I see here I think you have atrophied hands." And yes, he reported that he did. We are able to provide this type of information to people during Happy Hour. It is our way of giving back to the community.

Biofrequencies and Parkinsons Disease

If you want us to do the analysis for you, either join us on Happy Hour or call the office to set up a private appointment. Alternatively, you can take the training and learn how to do it yourself. That's what the Guardian Network is about. We meet once a month and go over what's happening.

One of the big things that we developed recently is a program called Radical Exposure. We had to change the name which used to be called Radiation Exposure because the FDA doesn't want anybody doing anything about radiation. This program allows people to know at a cellular level if they have cesium or uranium or plutonium that could be the cause of their symptoms.

There are nutritional antidotes and also competitor antidotes that will address radiation exposures. We look at the MathWays in the body which is the new system of BioAcoustic Biology. For example, if you have been exposed to strontium, the antidote is Adenosine Triphosphate. You can buy that over the counter at your local health food store. Choline is a competitor to strontium. People can purchase things that are the antidotes (or the competitors). So there are ways that people can do this on their own. If you are threatened with strontium - if strontium is in your water system - then you can look up the antidote that is shown on charts that are available to the public.

> **How can bio-frequencies help with detoxing heavy metals?**

SHARRY EDWARDS: We do it in two ways. We know what frequencies make the heavy metals give up their receptor site. You can do it with herbs but you can also do is using adenosine triphosphate (ATP). That's the first chemical made when conception takes place. It's the same frequency as white light and it really takes care of the body in a very positive way. It

Biofrequencies and Parkinsons Disease

also helps produce energy. It will bind heavy toxic metals including these radiation metals. You have to be really careful and watch for any kidney issues.

One of the stories that Marian told me is the doctor gave her something that really messed her up. She was able to watch her vocal print and fix herself from what the regular doctor had done to her.

MARIAN LEWIS: Right. It made my heart go crazy. I thought I was going to end up in the hospital because I knew this stuff was too strong for me. I was able to give myself the antidote and bring myself back to normal.

I did a vocal print a couple of times a day just to watch it and I could see what was happening. I was also taking my blood pressure and my pulse because my heart rate became very erratic. It really was very scary. By the time you call the doctor and they get to somebody and they get back to you to maybe make the change, you have to go get blood work and then they'll agree to change it. I told them all along it was too strong, but they wouldn't take my word for it of course. By that time I was fixing myself. They said, "Yes, you're right. It is way too strong." And then it will take six weeks for it to work. Well you know, I would've been dead by then. But it's much better now and improving every day with a lower dosage of medication and routinely watching my vocal print.

SHARRY EDWARDS: We're going to do a week long class just for Parkinson's and include a module on radiation. We will likely also cover the topics of methylation, allergies, Parkinson's, dystonia, spasticity, inflammation and even nutrition.

What can people do to get relief from their symptoms?

SHARRY EDWARDS: Get away from aspartame, get away from MSG, get away from gluten and avoid eating GMO

Biofrequencies and Parkinsons Disease

(genetically modified) products. There's an article about GMOs and cell signaling and how that's related to Parkinson's that's on our website under "research articles."

What do the tones sound like?

MARIAN LEWIS: It is not some kind of healing music that you can buy on a CD. It is not music. They are very low sounds. It sounds something like the fan running or the refrigerator running in the background.

The tones that are programmed will only support you. I can't hand over the tones that have been programmed for me for use by other people with Parkinson's symptoms.

SHARRY EDWARDS: The tones emulate the frequencies of your brain. Your brain speaks math: zero to 64 cycles per second. If we want to talk to your brain then we are going to speak math because that is the language your brain speaks. Math

Biofrequencies and Parkinsons Disease

can be defined using frequency.

MARIAN LEWIS: If you cup your hands over your ears you can hear the sounds of your body.

SHARRY EDWARDS: That sound is a form of feedback called an otoacoustic emission that is a perfect sound for you all you all time. It's a feedback loop of how our body is supposed to heal itself. We get into this in the class - all of this ancient stuff- and how to teach people to do it for themselves. That is what we really like to do - teach everybody to do this for themselves

MARIAN LEWIS: You can give somebody the wrong sounds and make them sicker, so that's why you need the training. You need to know what you're doing.

SHARRY EDWARDS: Absolutely and Marian's very responsive to sounds. You get ten seconds on her before she says "No, that's the wrong one, I don't want that."

MARIAN LEWIS: I'm just a super-sensitive chick.

SHARRY EDWARDS: You can make people strong or weak. You see people open up. They can't walk and now they can. They are in pain and now they aren't. It is beyond words to get to see that.

Marian, is your husband still a skeptic?

MARIAN LEWIS: Oh, he said today, "Don't you want to do my vocal print?" I said, "Really?" Yes, he's a faithful listener. If he has an issue, he comes to me. He said, "You want to do more testing?" I haven't really had the proper testing equipment yet. I have been working with our tones just using a tone box so it's much more difficult to do. The testing equipment finally arrived late this afternoon. We're having a great time and he's been very, very supportive. He has been doing housework. He's been cooking and this is not his thing. We're married

56 years and this is a miracle in itself, I tell you! He has just been great!

What does he say about the movement and the change in your face?

MARIAN LEWIS: He says, "You look good today." I don't know if he's afraid to say too much because he really isn't that expressive of a person, but I think he's afraid that maybe it will go away and then I'll be disappointed or something, I don't know. So he just keeps watching me and says, "Well, you know, you look like you did when you were in high school" or something like that. Now you know that we met when we were 16, so he has known me a long time.

SHARRY EDWARDS: That is the beauty of doing this with frequency and doing it individually. You take care of the first layer and then if it stops working you work with the second layer and so forth. It is not like when dopamine quits working because you got too used to it.

Biofrequencies and Parkinsons Disease

Your body will tell you every day what's the new thing that you need and you renew that.

MARIAN LEWIS: And it does change so you have to stay on top of it. I thank you both, you are both a gift, and without Dr. Rodgers I wouldn't have met Sharry. I feel you've given me and my whole family a new lease on life. I'm just grateful and I thank God for you every day.

SHARRY EDWARDS: Well, when you're 104 we'll allow you to quit teaching and talking about this.

MARIAN LEWIS: I told my son, I want to go to Disney World when I'm 100 and ride in the Mickey Mouse Parade. He'll only be about 80 and he can go with me.

SHARRY EDWARDS: The other software program that we have that a lot of people are excited about is the rejuvenation one which is the anti-aging. Marian can tell you I do not look like I'm 65 years old.

Biofrequencies and Parkinsons Disease

And people can go back and pick up that software when they become members and get a whole collection of all these different programs.

One free program that people can start their own practice with is called NanoVoice which can be downloaded from http://www.NanoVoice.org. There are instruction booklets (including instructions for Mac users) and some charts. That is our gift to the world because we want people to know that the frequencies of their voice tell other people who they are. You punch a few buttons and it spits out a report of who you are and how you're feeling for the day. When people see that, they realize their voice really does contain information that provides data about who they are and their state of health. It opens a whole new world to them.

MARIAN LEWIS: I tell my friends this really isn't a new thing. You already know *how to do this. When you call someone on the phone that you know pretty well and you'll say, "Oh, you're not having a good day today, are you?" You can tell by the sound of the voice. Or you're having a happy day or sad day or you're depressed or you're sick. It is all there in the voice. You know that over the phone. You can't see them, but you hear it in the voice so you already know all this.*

SHARRY EDWARDS: I think people intuitively know about this idea because they experience it as they are growing up. Think about young men going through puberty. Their voice changes in reaction to hormones. People experience that hormones change the voice, so why is it such a great leap to think that the frequencies of the voice could be used to glean information about protein and enzymes and so on? We cracked the codes for the genes and toxins and diseases and syndromes and nutrients and created a system of BioAcoustic Biology. My rose-

colored wish for the world is I want everybody to have this and if I had my way, and if I had enough money, I'd give it all away. But somebody's got to pay the light bill.

How could bio-frequencies do anything for a person with a gene that's defective?

SHARRY EDWARDS: We can help a person shut off or turn on a gene. The way that Dr. John Apsley became familiar with my work is that he was working with a little girl named April that had Downs Syndrome. She came here with her mother. April's symptoms, the face the large forehead, the slanted eyes, clubbed-looking fingers – all of it disappeared because we were able to shut down that gene.

MARIAN LEWIS: It's all frequency, your whole body, everything is made of frequency.

SHARRY EDWARDS: Absolutely. Frequency comes first and then the body *manifests. Go to <u>You Tube</u> and search my name, Sharry Edwards. Note that Sharry is spelled with an "a". You can see videos that show the reversal of stroke damage, regeneration of the voice, reversal of MS, restructuring of somebody's leg that was in a state of trauma, bringing some people out of comas, getting rid of back pain, getting rid of tumors, getting rid of epilepsy... It's all there and it's all documented.*

The bio-frequency technology allows you to see the disease process before it is manifested. You can see it beforehand. We can look at cancer before it ever happens. You can look at vitamin A frequencies go very high, <u>catalase</u> frequencies go very low and that <u>calcitonin</u> which controls the calcium of the body begins to be unbalanced. In looking at those three, people can tell years ahead of time what is going on with their body. Catalase helps the body get rid of fluid debris from the body. Vitamin A *helps support antioxidant activity, helps support biosalts and the helps support use of beta carotene.*

Here is what happens to the body. I'm not making this up; this comes from Dr. Robert O. Becker. When the body gets traumatized or hurt or cut, the cells send out a "rescue me" signal and that calls calcium to the site. When there is no calcium, there is a cancer food in the body that is 1/100th different from the frequency of calcium. If there is no calcium in the system, it is our theory that the body calls to it this frequency and it is food for cancer.

If people with a history of cancer in their families keep their calcium levels up and running and maintain necessary levels of calcitonin (which is a regulator of calcium in the blood) it is doubtful they are going to have to go ahead and experience the cancer. That is an incredibly profound piece of information that ought to be universally known.

There are other things that happen but this is one of the most important. It is called 5-HETE and it is a cancer food. It creates itself out of a fault involving arachidonic acid and hydrogen peroxide and that is in the actual medical literature. But we can watch it by way of its frequencies in the body.

Here is another piece about cancer that sort of ticks me off. They (the medical research community) have known for years that chronic lymphocytic leukemia is associated with the inability of the body to process cortisol. I have found that in the literature in an article written in 1929 – nobody had listened to this guy – and when the body begins not to be able to use cortisol, leukemia can manifest because the body just can't replenish the cells that are dying faster than the body can replenish or fight off whatever is attacking.

Now, if they've known that for this many years, why don't they use it? Have you ever heard of cortisol being used in the fight of cancer? Not likely. But we can look at iron, we can look at the iron molecule (in terms of frequency), we can look at what is going on with chronic lymphocytic leukemia, look at their cortisol and balance it by providing the biofrequencies indicated by their vocal print. I don't know if you can buy cortisol off the shelf but we can provide it to people by sound, but we do it all experimentally.

Is there a connection between tetanus inoculations and Parkinson's symptoms?

SHARRY EDWARDS: Absolutely. Especially if you've got problems with the little toe side of the foot; there is either pain there or that side of the foot is curling under, then it is usually the live tetanus virus that is causing it. And lockjaw, it looks like Parkinson's. People experience the feeling of muscle freeze a lot. They try to take a step and the muscles just won't behave. They won't go where they ought to go. It is really tetanus and they're not willing to admit that there are vaccination relationships that are going on with Parkinson's symptoms. Marian had that in her chart and some of her toes turning under. We had to give her the antidote for the tetanus shot.

MARIAN LEWIS: Yes, and it straightened out in a very short time.

SHARRY EDWARDS: We can kill pathogens with this. We can open receptor sites. You may have your receptor site for GABA closed down and you may experience Bi-polar symptoms because of that. We can help the body open that receptor site or close it. We can help support a gene, but some things that are really high in the voice we don't want to mess with.

Biofrequencies and Parkinsons Disease

If you have a longevity gene and it is high and off the chart, who cares, right? If you have a pathogen gene and it is very low, who cares if a pathogen frequency's low? We don't want it to be high. So you have to use some common sense with all of this and that's what we teach in the week-long class.

People can go ahead and join the once-a-month class and get their toes wet and see if this is what they'd like to do, or they can join us for Happy Hour every other Tuesday and watch it happen. This is so easy; I don't know why somebody didn't do this eons ago. It makes sense. You've got an energy body. Let's find out what makes the energy body work. Let's put it back into perfect balance and ta-da! Perfect health.

We want to do a pre-class just for the Parkinson's. We'll put it up on You Tube or on your site so people can come in and look at how to use these programs, then we'll plan the week-long course. And people can do it online. They don't have to come here. They are welcome to, but they can do all of it without leaving their computer chair. There are cameras so you can watch what we're doing

MARIAN LEWIS: There is 'sound hope,' people; there is 'sound hope'! Even though it's online, people need to understand that they help you every step of the way and you can ask a million questions like I do and they always answer them, so you don't need to feel alone.

How to Hear Marian Lewis and Sharry Edwards on Parkinsons Recovery Radio

Visit http://www.blogtalkradio.com/parkinsons-recovery and scroll back to find the show that aired August 31, 2011 featuring Sharry Edwards and Marian Lewis as my guests.

About Sharry Edwards

Sharry Edwards is the pioneer in the study of Human BioAcoustic Biology.

Her 30 years of research is being used at the Institute of BioAcoustic Biology in Albany, OH. Currently, Edwards and her team at Sound Health are using the human voice and the

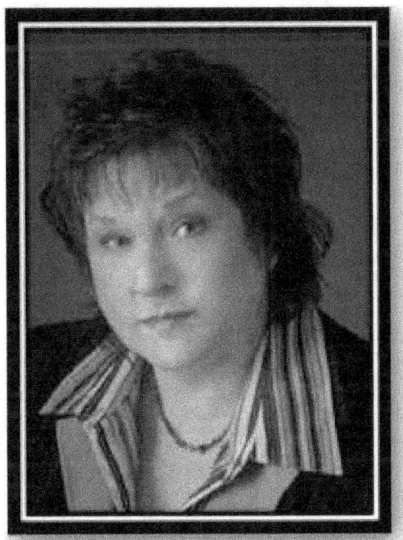

associated frequencies to help clients with Parkinsons Disease in addition to many other chronic illnesses.

Sharry Edwards' work is now included in The Duke University Encyclopedia of New Medicine, by Leonard A. Wisnecki and The Scientific Basis of Integrative Medicine, by Lucy Anderson. The effects of BioAcoustic Biology, now accepted by these prestigious medical encyclopedias,

Biofrequencies and Parkinsons Disease

have unlimited health and wellness
potential.

According to Edwards, "BioAcoustics
Voice Spectral Analysis can detect
hidden or underlying stresses in the
body that are expressed as disease."
Vocal prints can identify toxins,
pathogens and nutritional
supplements that are too low or too
high. In addition, vocal prints can be
used to match the most compatible
treatment remedy to each client. The
introduction of the proper low
frequency sound to the body,
indicated through voice analysis, has
been shown to help people who
currently experience the symptoms of
Parkinsons Disease. Sharry can be
contacted at:
SharryEdwards@gmail.com

About Marian Lewis

Being born a Southwestern
Pennsylvania coal miner's daughter

and eldest of five children, Marian learned to sew out of necessity at a very early age. Teaching others her common sense techniques became her passion that helped to support her family for more than fifty years. She lectured and wrote sewing articles and published eBooks' on sewing and fitting all without any formal training. With her grandchildren's urging, Marian researched the family history and wrote a five generation family cookbook to help preserve so many family traditions.

She married her high school sweetheart; has a son and daughter and two grandsons and two granddaughters – all of whom she and her husband of 55 years are very proud.

Both Marian and her husband are cancer survivors (two and three times each) and have lost many friends and

family members to this disease that

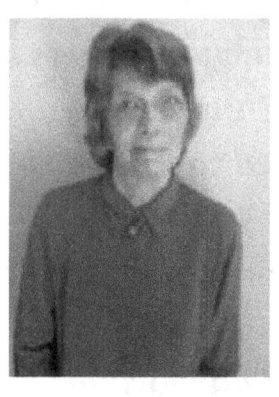

they believe was caused by exposure to radioactive material many years ago in their community. It was the worst disaster east of the Mississippi that very few people ever knew about.

Having a strong faith and will to survive, Marian approached Parkinson's Disease at age 72 with the same fervor. Not able to tolerate drugs very well with her sensitive immune system, Marian sought other therapies to help alleviate her symptoms. She feels that she is "on the road to recovery" using Sound Health bio acoustic therapy offered by Sharry Edwards. Even with this disease and her age of 74, Marian is determined to move forward. She recently took the training to become a

BioAcoustic Research Associate (BARA) not only to help herself and family, but to offer sound hope to so many other Parkinson people in SW Florida where she now resides. This is only the beginning concerning her incredible journey to wellness. Contact Marian at:

mailto:marian.lewis56@gmail.com